Anti-Inflammatory Diet Meal Plan 2021

30 Days Meal Plans with Tasty Recipes to Heal
the Immune System and Reducing Inflammation

Joy Sanford

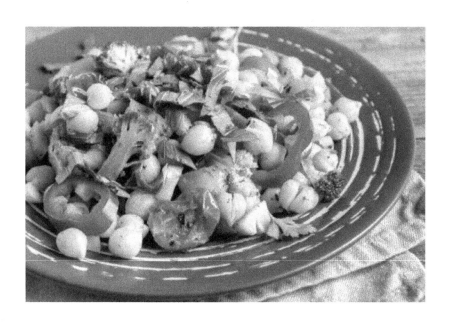

Table of Contents

the publisher or the original author of this work can be in any fashion deemed liable for any hardship or damages that may befall them after undertaking information described herein. Additionally, the information in the following pages is intended only for informational purposes and should thus be thought of as universal. As befitting its nature, it is presented without assurance regarding its prolonged validity or interim quality. Trademarks that are mentioned are done without written consent and can in no way be considered an endorsement from the trademark holder.

Introduction

Most of the widely consumed diets incorporate anti-inflammation diet principles. In particular, the Mediterranean diet has whole grains, fish, and fats that are beneficial for the heart. Studies suggest that this diet can help lower the effects of cardiovascular system inflammation due to diet. Taking an anti-inflammatory diet is can be a complementary therapy for most conditions that are aggravated by chronic inflammation.

An anti-inflammation diet entails eating only particular kinds of food and avoiding others to lower the symptoms of chronic inflammatory diseases. It is one of the recommended measures that an individual can take to reduce or prevent inflammation induced by diet.

Expectedly, an anti-inflammatory diet involves nutrient-dense plant foods and minimizing or avoiding processed meats and foods. The goal of an anti-inflammation diet is to minimize inflammatory responses. The diet entails substituting refined foods with whole and nutrient-laden foods. Predictably, an anti-inflammation diet will contain more amounts of antioxidants that are reactive molecules in food and help reduce the number of free radicals. The free radicals are molecules in the human body that may harm cells and enhance the risk of certain diseases.

In particular, an anti-inflammation diet can help with the following diseases/conditions:

- Diabetes

Focusing exclusively on type 2 diabetes arises when the body fails to properly utilize insulin leading to higher than normal blood sugar levels. The condition of more sugar levels in the blood than normal is also known as hyperglycemia. It is also called insulin resistance. At the beginning of type 2 diabetes, the pancreas tries to make more insulin but fails to catch up with the rising blood sugar levels.

- Inflammatory bowel disease

Inflammatory bowel disease is a common gastrointestinal disorder that affects the large intestine. The symptoms of inflammatory bowel disease include abdominal pain, cramping, bloating, constipation, and diarrhea. It is a chronic condition, and it has to be managed in the long-term. Dietary measures are necessary to prevent diet-induced bloating, abdominal pain, diarrhea, and constipation. However, only a small percentage of individuals with inflammatory bowel disease will have extreme symptoms manifestation.

- Obesity

Medically, obesity refers to a complex disorder involving excessive amounts of body fat. Expectedly, obesity increases the risk of heart diseases as well as other health problems. Fortunately, modest weight loss can help halt and reverse the effects of obesity. Dietary adjustments can help address the causes of obesity, and the anti-inflammatory diet is inherently a healthy diet.

· Heart disease

Cardiovascular diseases can be triggered by diet, and diet can is used to manage several heart diseases. Food-related factors that increase the risk of heart diseases include obesity and high blood pressure. The type of fat eaten can also worsen or lesser risk of developing heart disease. In particular, cholesterol, saturated and trans fats are thought to increase heart attack rates. Most obese individuals also tend to have high-fat diets.

• Metabolic syndrome

Medically, metabolic syndrome refers to a group of factors that manifest together, leading to an increase in the risk of developing other inflammatory conditions. Some of these conditions include high blood pressure, excess body fat, especially around the waist, abnormal cholesterol, and high blood sugar levels. Having any or all of these conditions signifies that you are at a higher risk of developing a chronic condition. Most of these conditions are also associated with consuming an inflammation diet.

• Hashimoto's disease

Hashimoto's disease is an autoimmune disorder in which the body attacks its own tissues and, in particular, the thyroid organ. The result of unmanaged Hashimoto's disease is hypothyroidism implying that the body will not make adequate hormones. The thyroid gland makes hormones that control body metabolism, which includes heart rate and calories utilization. Unchecked Hashimoto's disease will also result in difficulties in swallowing when goiter manifests. Diet adjustments can be used to help manage the disease along with medications.

• Lupus

Lupus is another autoimmune disease that occurs when the body attacks its own organs and tissues. The inflammation occasioned by unmanaged lupus will affect other parts of the body. For instance, inflammation triggered by lupus will affect the heart, lungs, kidneys, and skin, including the brain and blood cells. The common symptoms of lupus are fever, fatigue, chest pain, dry eyes, and butterfly-shaped rash. Diet can be used to minimize the worsening of inflammation by adhering to the anti-inflammatory diet.

The other benefit of taking an anti-inflammation diet is that it can help lower the risk of select cancers such as colorectal cancer.

30 Days Meal Plan

Days	Breakfast	Lunch	Dinner	Snacks/desserts
1	Carrot Cake Overnight Oats	Strawberries and Cream Trifle	Pan-Seared Halibut with Citrus Butter Sauce	Candied Dates
2	Mediterranean Frittata	Maple Toast and Eggs	Sole Asiago	Berry Delight
3	Maple Oatmeal	Sweet Onion and Egg Pie	Cheesy Garlic Salmon	Blueberry & Chia Flax Seed Pudding
4	Tomato Omelet	Mini Breakfast Pizza	Stuffed Chicken Breasts	Spicy Roasted chickpeas
5	Tuna & Sweet Potato	Chicken Muffins	Spicy Pork Chops	Berry Energy bites

	Croquette s			
6	Quinoa & Veggie Croquette s	Pumpkin Pancakes	Almond Breaded Chicken Goodness	Roasted Beets
7	Turkey Burgers	Cauliflo wer and Chorizo	Garlic Lamb Chops	Bruschetta
8	Salmon Burgers	Carrot Bread	Mushroo m Pork Chops	Cashew Cheese
9	Quinoa & Beans Burgers	Fruity Muffins	Mediterra nean Pork	Low Cholesterol- Low Calorie Blueberry Muffin
10	Veggie Balls	Edamam e Omelet	Brie- Packed Smoked Salmon	Carrot Sticks with Avocado Dip
11	Coconut & Banana Cookies	Almond Mascarp one	Blackened Tilapia	Boiled Okra and Squash

		Dumplings		
12	Fennel Seeds Cookies	Raisin Bran Muffins	Salsa Chicken Bites	Oven Crisp Sweet Potato
13	Almond Scones	Apple Bread	Tomato & Tuna Balls	Olive and Tomato Balls
14	Oven-Poached Eggs	Zucchini Bread	Fennel & Figs Lamb	Mini Pepper Nachos
15	Cranberry and Raisins Granola	Sweetened Brown Rice	Tamari Steak Salad	Avocado Hummus
16	Spicy Marble Eggs	Cornmeal Grits	Blackened Chicken	Flavorsome Almonds
17	Nutty Oats Pudding	Grapefruit-Pomegranate Salad	Mediterranean Mushroom Olive Steak	Chewy Blackberry Leather

18	Almond Pancakes with Coconut Flakes	Oatmeal-Raisin Scones	Buttery Scallops	Party-Time Chicken Nuggets
19	Bake Apple Turnover	Yogurt Cheese and Fruit	Brussels Sprouts and Garlic Aioli	Protein-Packed Croquettes
20	Quinoa and Cauliflower Congee	Chicken & Cabbage Platter	Broccoli Bites	Energy Dates Balls
21	Breakfast Arrozcaldo	Balsamic Chicken and Vegetables	Bacon Burger Cabbage Stir Fry	Energetic Oat Bars
22	Apple Bruschetta with Almonds and Blackberries	Onion Bacon Pork Chops	Bacon Cheeseburger	Soft Flourless Cookies

23	Hash Browns	Caramelized Pork Chops	Cauliflower Mac & Cheese	Delectable Cookies
24	Sun-Dried Tomato Garlic Bruschetta	Chicken Bacon Quesadilla	Mushroom & Cauliflower Risotto	Turmeric Chickpea Cakes
25	Mushroom Crêpes	Sesame-Crusted Tuna with Green Beans	Pita Pizza	Almonds and Blueberries Yogurt Snack
26	Oat Porridge with Cherry & Coconut	Rosemary Roasted Pork with Cauliflower	Skillet Cabbage Tacos	Peanut Butter and Honey Oat Bars
27	Gingerbread Oatmeal Breakfast	Grilled Salmon and Zucchini	Taco Casserole	Cottage Cheese with Apple Sauce

		with Mango Sauce		
28	Apple, Ginger, and Rhubarb Muffins	Beef and Broccoli Stir-Fry	Creamy Chicken Salad	Cucumber Rolls Hors D'oeuvres
29	Anti-Inflammatory Breakfast Frittata	Parmesan-Crusted Halibut with Asparagus	Spicy Keto Chicken Wings	Ginger Turmeric Protein Bars
30	Breakfast Sausage and Mushroom Casserole	Hearty Beef and Bacon Casserole	Cheesy Ham Quiche	Avocado with Tomatoes and Cucumber

Breakfast

Carrot Cake Overnight Oats

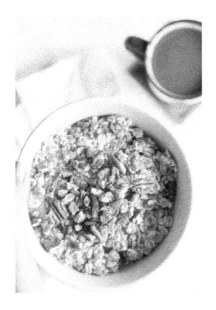

Preparation Time: 5 minutes + overnight

Cooking Time: 0 minutes

Servings: 1

Ingredients:

1. 1 cup Coconut or almond milk
2. 1 tbsp. Chia seeds
3. 1 tsp. Cinnamon, ground
4. ½ cup Raisins

5. 2 tbsp. Cream cheese, low fat, at room temperature
6. 1 Large Carrot, peel, and shred
7. 2 tbsp. Honey
8. 1 tsp. Vanilla

Directions:

- Mix together all of the listed ingredients and store them in a safe refrigerator container overnight. Eat cold in the morning. If you choose to warm this, just microwave for one minute and stir well before eating.

Nutrition:

Calories 340

32 grams sugar

8 grams protein

4 grams fat

9 grams fiber

70 grams carbs

Mediterranean Frittata

Preparation Time: 5 minutes

Cooking Time: 20 minutes

Servings: 6

Ingredients:

1. 6 Eggs
2. ¼ cup Feta cheese, crumbled
3. ¼ tsp. Black pepper
4. Oil, spray or olive
5. 1 tsp. Oregano
6. ¼ cup Milk, almond or coconut
7. 1 tsp. Sea salt
8. ¼ cup Black olives, chopped
9. ¼ cup Green olives, chopped
10. ¼ cup Tomatoes, diced

Directions:

- Heat oven to 400. Oil one eight by eight-inch baking dish. Beat the milk into the eggs, and then add other ingredients. Pour all of this mixture into the baking dish and bake for twenty minutes.

Nutrition: Calories 107

2 grams sugars

7 fat grams,3 carb grams,7 grams protein

Maple Oatmeal

Preparation Time: 5 minutes

Cooking Time: 20 minutes

Servings: 4

Ingredients:

1. 1 tsp. Maple flavoring
2. 1 tsp. Cinnamon
3. 3 tbsp. Sunflower seeds
4. ½ cup Pecans, chopped
5. ¼ cup Coconut flakes, unsweetened
6. ½ cup Walnuts, chopped
7. ½ cup Milk, almond or coconut
8. 4 tbsp. Chia seeds

Directions:

- Pulse the sunflower seeds, walnuts, and pecans in a food processor to crumble. Or you can just put the nuts in a sturdy plastic bag, wrap the bag with a towel, lay it on a sturdy surface, and beat the towel with a hammer until the nuts are crumbled. Mix the crushed nuts with the rest of the ingredients and pour them into a large pot. Simmer this mixture over low heat for thirty minutes. Stir often, so the mix does not stick to the bottom. Serve garnished with fresh fruit or a sprinkle of cinnamon if desired.

Nutrition:

Calories 374

3.2 grams carbs

9.25 grams protein

34.59 grams fat

Tomato Omelet

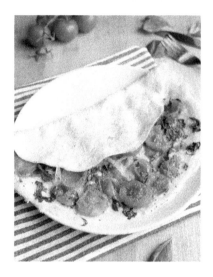

Preparation Time: 2 minutes

Cooking Time: 8 minutes

Servings: 1

Ingredients:

1. 2 Eggs
2. ½ cup Basil, fresh
3. ½ cup Cherry tomatoes
4. 1 tsp. Black pepper
5. ¼ cup Cheese, any type, shredded
6. ½ tsp. Salt
7. 2 tbsp. Olive oil

Directions:

1. Cut the tomatoes into quarters. Fry the tomatoes for 3 hours. Set the tomatoes off to the side. Add the salt and pepper to the eggs in a small bowl and beat together well. Pour the mix of beaten egg into the pan and use a spatula to gently work around the edges under the omelet, letting the eggs fry unmoved for three minutes. When just the center third of the egg mix is still runny, add on the basil, tomatoes, and cheese. Fold over half of the omelet onto the other half. Cook two more minutes and serve.

Nutrition:

Calories 342

8 grams carbs

20 grams protein

25.3 grams fat

Tuna & Sweet Potato Croquettes

Preparation Time: 15 minutes

Cooking Time: 12 minutes

Servings: 8

Ingredients:

- 1 tablespoon coconut oil
- ½ large onion, chopped
- 1 (1-inch piece fresh ginger, minced
- 3 garlic cloves, minced
- 1 Serrano pepper, seeded and minced
- ½ teaspoon ground coriander
- ¼ teaspoon ground turmeric
- ¼ teaspoon red chili powder
- ¼ teaspoon garam masala
- Salt, to taste
- Freshly ground black pepper, to taste
- 2 (5 oz.) cans tuna
- 1 cup sweet potato, peeled and mashed
- 1 egg
- ¼ cup tapioca flour
- ¼ cup almond flour
- Olive oil, as required

Directions:

2. In a frying pan, warm the coconut oil on medium heat.
3. Put onion, ginger, garlic, and Serrano pepper and sauté for approximately 5-6 minutes.
4. Stir in spices and sauté approximately 1 minute more.
5. Transfer the onion mixture in a bowl.
6. Add tuna and sweet potato and mix till well combined.
7. Make equal sized oblong shaped patties in the mixture.
8. Arrange the croquettes inside a baking sheet in a very single layer and refrigerate for overnight.
9. In a shallow dish, beat the egg.
10. In another shallow dish, mix together both flours.
11. In a big skillet, heat the enough oil.
12. Add croquettes in batches and shallow fry for around 2-3 minutes per side.

Nutrition:

Calories: 404

Fat: 9g

Carbohydrates: 20g

Fiber: 4g

Protein: 30g

Quinoa & Veggie Croquettes

Preparation Time: 15 minutes

Cooking Time: 9 minutes

Servings: 12-15

Ingredients:

1. 1 tbsp. essential olive oil
2. ½ cup frozen peas, thawed
3. 2 minced garlic cloves
4. 1 cup cooked quinoa
5. 2 large boiled potatoes, peeled and mashed
6. ¼ cup fresh cilantro leaves, chopped
7. 2 teaspoons ground cumin
8. 1 teaspoon garam masala
9. ¼ teaspoon ground turmeric
10. Salt, to taste
11. Freshly ground black pepper, to taste
12. Olive oil, for frying

Directions:

- In a frying pan, warm oil on medium heat.
- Add peas and garlic and sauté for about 1 minute.
- Transfer the pea mixture into a large bowl.
- Add the remainder ingredients and mix till well combined.

- Make equal sized oblong shaped patties from your mixture.
- In a huge skillet, heat oil on medium-high heat.
- Add croquettes and fry for about 4 minutes per side.

Nutrition:

Calories: 367

Fat: 6g

Carbohydrates: 17g

Fiber: 5g

Protein: 22g

Turkey Burgers

Preparation Time: 15 minutes

Cooking Time: 8 minutes

Servings: 5

Ingredients:

- 1 ripe pear, peeled, cored and chopped roughly
- 1-pound lean ground turkey
- 1 teaspoon fresh ginger, grated finely
- 2 minced garlic cloves
- 1 teaspoon fresh rosemary, minced
- 1 teaspoon fresh sage, minced
- Salt, to taste
- Freshly ground black pepper, to taste
- 1-2 tablespoons coconut oil

Directions:

- In a blender, add pear and pulse till smooth.
- Transfer the pear mixture in a large bowl with remaining ingredients except for oil and mix till well combined.
- Make small equal sized 10 patties from the mixture.
- In a heavy-bottomed frying pan, heat oil on medium heat.

- Add the patties and cook for around 4-5 minutes.
- Flip the inside and cook for approximately 2-3 minutes.

Nutrition:

Calories: 477

Fat: 15g

Carbohydrates: 26g

Fiber: 11g

Protein: 35g

Salmon Burgers

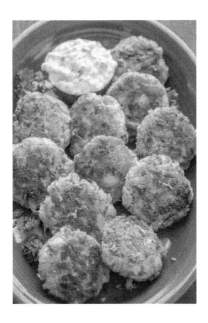

Preparation Time: 15 minutes

Cooking Time: 8 minutes

Servings: 3

Ingredients:

1. 1 (6-oz. can) skinless, boneless salmon, drained
2. 1 celery rib, chopped
3. ½ of a medium onion, chopped
4. 2 large eggs
5. 1 tablespoon plus 1 teaspoon coconut flour
6. 1 tablespoon dried dill, crushed
7. 1 teaspoon lemon
8. Salt, to taste

9. Freshly ground black pepper, to taste
10. 3 tablespoons coconut oil

Directions:

1. In a substantial bowl, add salmon and which has a fork, break it into small pieces.
2. Add remaining ingredients excluding the for oil and mix till well combined.
3. Make 6 equal sized small patties from the mixture.
4. In a substantial skillet, melt coconut oil on medium-high heat.
5. Cook the patties for around 3-4 minutes per side.

Nutrition:

Calories: 393
Fat: 12g
Carbohydrates: 19g
Fiber: 5g
Protein: 24g

Quinoa & Beans Burgers

Preparation Time: 15 minutes

Cooking Time: 55 minutes

Servings: 12

Ingredients:

1. ½ cup dry quinoa
2. 1½ cups water
3. 1 cup cooked corn kernels
4. 1 (15 oz.) can black beans, drained
5. 1 small boiled potato, peeled
6. 1 small onion, chopped
7. ½ teaspoon fresh ginger, grated finely
8. 1 teaspoon garlic, minced
9. ½ cup fresh cilantro, chopped
10. 1 teaspoon flax meal
11. 1 teaspoon ground cumin
12. 1 teaspoon paprika
13. 1 teaspoon chili flakes
14. ½ teaspoon ground turmeric
15. Salt, to taste
16. Freshly ground black pepper, to taste

Directions:

- In a pan, add water and quinoa on high heat and provide to a boil.

- Lower the heat to medium and simmer for around 15-twenty or so minutes.
- Drain excess water.
- Set the oven to 375°F. Line a sizable baking sheet that has a parchment paper.
- In a sizable bowl, add quinoa and remaining ingredients.
- With a fork, mix till well combined.
- Make equal-sized patties from the mixture.
- Arrange the patties onto the prepared baking sheet in the single layer.
- Bake for around 20-25 minutes.
- Carefully, alter the side and cook for about 8-10 minutes.

Nutrition:

Calories: 400

Fat: 9g

Carbohydrates: 27g

Fiber: 12g

Protein: 38g

Veggie Balls

Preparation Time: 15 minutes

Cooking Time: 25 minutes

Servings: 5-6

Ingredients:

1. 2 medium sweet potatoes, cubed into ½-inch size
2. 2 tablespoons coconut milk
3. 1 cup fresh kale leaves, trimmed and chopped
4. 1 medium shallot, chopped finely
5. 1 tsp. ground cumin
6. ½ teaspoon granulated garlic
7. ¼ tsp. ground turmeric
8. Salt, to taste
9. Freshly ground black pepper, to taste

Ground flax seeds, as required

Directions:

- Set the oven to 400°F. Line a baking sheet with parchment paper.
- In a pan of water, arrange a steamer basket.
- Bring the sweet potato in a steamer basket and steam approximately 10-15 minutes.
- In a sizable bowl, put the sweet potato.
- Add coconut milk and mash well.

- Add remaining ingredients except for flax seeds and mix till well combined.
- Make about 1½-2-inch balls from your mixture.
- Arrange the balls onto the prepared baking sheet inside a single layer.
- Sprinkle with flax seeds.
- Bake for around 20-25 minutes.

Nutrition:

Calories: 464

Fat: 12g

Carbohydrates: 20g

Fiber: 8g

Protein: 27g

Coconut & Banana Cookies

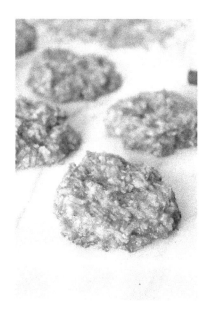

Preparation Time: 15 minutes

Cooking Time: 25 minutes

Servings: 7

Ingredients:

1. 2 cups unsweetened coconut, shredded
2. 3 medium bananas, peeled
3. ½ tsp. ground cinnamon
4. ½ tsp. ground turmeric
5. Pinch of salt, to taste
6. Freshly ground black pepper

Directions:

- Set the oven to 350°F. Line a cookie sheet a lightly greased parchment paper.
- In a mixer, put all together ingredients and pulse till a dough-like mixture forms.
- Form small balls through the mixture and set onto a prepared cookie sheet in a single layer.
- Using your fingers, press along the balls to create the cookies.
- Bake for at least 15-20 minutes or till golden brown.

Nutrition:

Calories: 370

Fat: 4g

Carbohydrates: 28g

Fiber: 11g

Protein: 33g

Fennel Seeds Cookies

Preparation Time: 10 minutes

Cooking Time: 20 minutes

Servings: 5

Ingredients:

- 1/3 cup coconut flour
- ¼ teaspoon whole fennel seeds
- ½ teaspoon fresh ginger, grated finely
- ¼ cup coconut oil, softened
- 2 tablespoons raw honey
- 1 teaspoon vanilla extract
- Pinch of ground cinnamon
- Pinch of salt
- Pinch freshly ground black pepper

Directions:

1. Set the oven to 360°F. Line a cookie sheet that has a parchment paper.
2. In a substantial bowl, add all together the ingredients and mix till an even dough form.
3. Form a small balls in the mixture make onto a prepared cookie sheet inside a single layer.
4. Using your fingers, gently press along the balls to create the cookies.
5. Bake for at least 9 minutes or till golden brown.

Nutrition:

Calories: 353

Fat: 5g

Carbohydrates: 19g

Fiber: 3g

Protein: 25g

Almond Scones

Preparation Time: 10 minutes

Cooking Time: 20 minutes

Servings: 6

Ingredients:

- 1 cup almonds
- 1 1/3 cups almond flour
- ¼ cup arrowroot flour
- 1 tablespoon coconut flour
- 1 teaspoon ground turmeric
- Salt, to taste
- Freshly ground black pepper, to taste
- 1 egg
- ¼ cup essential olive oil
- 3 tablespoons raw honey
- 1 teaspoon vanilla flavoring

Directions:

- In a mixer, put almonds then pulse till chopped roughly
- Move the chopped almonds in a big bowl.
- Put flours and spices and mix well.
- In another bowl, put the remaining ingredients and beat till well combined.

- Put the flour mixture into the egg mixture then mix till well combined.
- Arrange a plastic wrap over the cutting board.
- Place the dough over the cutting board.
- Using both of your hands, pat into 1-inch thick circle.
- Cut the circle in 6 wedges.
- Set the scones onto a cookie sheet in a single layer.
- Bake for at least 15-20 minutes.

Nutrition:

Calories: 304

Fat: 3g

Carbohydrates: 22g

Fiber: 6g

Protein: 20g

Oven-Poached Eggs

Preparation Time: 2minutes

Cooking Time: 11minutes

Servings: 4

Ingredients:

- 6 eggs, at room temperature
- Water
- Ice bath
- 2 cups water, chilled
- 2 cups of ice cubes

Directions:

1. Set the oven to 350°F. Put 2 cups of water into a deep roasting tin, and place it into the lowest rack of the oven.
2. Place one egg into each cup of cupcake/muffin tins, along with one tablespoon of water.
3. Carefully place muffin tins into the middle rack of the oven.
4. Bake eggs for 45 minutes.
5. Turn off the heat immediately. Take off the muffin tins from the oven and set on a cake rack to cool before extracting eggs.
6. Pour ice bath ingredients into a large heat-resistant bowl.

7. Bring the eggs into an ice bath to stop the cooking process. After 10 minutes, drain eggs well. Use as needed.

Nutrition:

Calories: 357 kcal

Protein: 17.14 g

Fat: 24.36 g

Carbohydrates: 16.19 g

Cranberry and Raisins Granola

Preparation Time: 15 minutes

Cooking Time: 20 minutes

Servings: 4

Ingredients:

- 4 cups old-fashioned rolled oats
- 1/4 cup sesame seeds
- 1 cup dried cranberries
- 1 cup golden raisins
- 1/8 teaspoon nutmeg
- 2 tablespoons olive oil
- 1/2 cup almonds, slivered
- 2 tablespoons warm water
- 1 teaspoon vanilla extract
- 1 teaspoon cinnamon
- 1/4 teaspoon of salt
- 6 tablespoons maple syrup
- 1/3 cup of honey

Directions:

1. In a bowl, mix the sesame seeds, nutmeg, almonds, oats, salt, and cinnamon.
2. In another bowl, mix the oil, water, vanilla, honey, and syrup. Gradually pour the mixture into the oats mixture. Toss to combine. Spread

the mixture into a greased jelly-roll pan. Bake in the oven at 300°F for at least 55 minutes. Stir and break the clumps every 10 minutes.

3. Once you get it from the oven, stir the cranberries and raisins. Allow cooling. This will last for a week when stored in an airtight container and up to a month when stored in the fridge.

Nutrition:

Calories: 698 kcal

Protein: 21.34 g

Fat: 20.99 g

Carbohydrates: 148.59 g

Spicy Marble Eggs

Preparation Time: 15 minutes

Cooking Time: 2 hours

Servings: 12

Ingredients:

1. 6 medium-boiled eggs, unpeeled, cooled
2. For the Marinade
3. 2 oolong black tea bags
4. 3 Tbsp. brown sugar
5. 1 thumb-sized fresh ginger, unpeeled, crushed
6. 3 dried star anise, whole
7. 2 dried bay leaves
8. 3 Tbsp. light soy sauce
9. 4 Tbsp. dark soy sauce
10. 4 cups of water
11. 1 dried cinnamon stick, whole
12. 1 tsp. salt
13. 1 tsp. dried Szechuan peppercorns

Directions:

- Using the back of a metal spoon, crack eggshells in places to create a spider web effect. Do not peel. Set aside until needed.

- Pour marinade into large Dutch oven set over high heat. Put lid partially on. Bring water to a rolling boil, about 5 minutes. Turn off heat.
- Secure lid. Steep ingredients for 10 minutes.
- Using a slotted spoon, fish out and discard solids. Cool marinade completely to room proceeding.
- Place eggs into an airtight non-reactive container just small enough to snugly fit all these in.
- Pour in marinade. Eggs should be completely submerged in liquid. Discard leftover marinade, if any. Line container rim with generous layers of saran wrap. Secure container lid.
- Chill eggs for 24 hours before using.
- Extract eggs and drain each piece well before using, but keep the rest submerged in the marinade.

Nutrition:
Calories: 75 kcal,Protein: 4.05 g, Fat: 4.36 g
Carbohydrates: 4.83 g

Nutty Oats Pudding

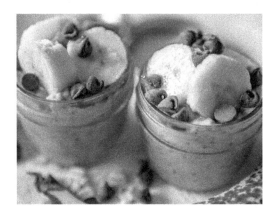

Preparation Time: 5 minutes

Cooking Time: 0 minutes

Servings: 3 -5

Ingredients:

1. ¼ cup rolled oats
2. 1 tablespoon yogurt, fat-free
3. 1 ½ tablespoon natural peanut butter
4. ¼ cup dry milk
5. 1 teaspoon peanuts, finely chopped
6. ½ cup of water

Directions:

- Using a microwaveable-safe bowl, put together peanut butter and dry milk. Whisk well. Add in water to achieve a smooth consistency. Add in oats.

- Cover bowl with plastic wrap. Create a small hole for the steam to escape.
- Place inside the microwave oven for 1 minute on high powder.
- Continue heating, this time on medium power for 90 seconds. Let sit for 5 minutes.
- To serve, spoon an equal amount of cereals in a bowl top with peanuts and yogurt.

Nutrition:

Calories: 70 kcal

Protein: 4.25 g

Fat: 3.83 g

Carbohydrates: 6.78 g

Almond Pancakes with Coconut Flakes

Preparation: Time: 5 minutes

Cooking Time: 10 minutes

Servings: 6

Ingredients:

1. 1 overripe banana, mashed
2. 2 eggs, yolks, and whites separated
3. ½ cup unsweetened applesauce
4. 1 cup almond flour, finely milled
5. ¼ cup of water
6. ¼ tsp. coconut oil
7. Garnish
8. 2 Tbsp. blanched almond flakes
9. Dash of cinnamon powder
10. ¼ cup coconut flakes, sweetened
11. Pinch of sea salt
12. Pure maple syrup, use sparingly

Directions:

- Whisk egg whites until soft peaks form.
- Except for egg whites and coconut oil, combine remaining ingredients in another bowl. Mix until batter comes together.

- Gently fold in egg whites. Make sure that you don't over mix, or the pancake will become dense and chewy.
- Pour oil into a nonstick skillet set over medium heat.
- Wait for the oil to heat up before dropping in approximately ½ cup of batter. Cook until each side are set, and bubbles form in the center. Turn on the other side then cook for another 2 minutes.
- Transfer flapjacks to a plate. Repeat step until all batter is cooked. Pour in more oil into the skillet only if needed. This recipe should yield between 4 to 6 medium-sized pancakes.
- Stack pancakes. Pour the desired amount of pure maple syrup on top. Garnish each stack with cinnamon-flavored almond-coconut flakes just before serving.
- For the garnish, set the oven to 350°F for at least 10 minutes before use. Line a baking sheet with parchment paper. Set aside.
- Mix almond and coconut flakes together in a bowl. Spread mixture evenly on a prepared baking sheet.

- Bake for 7 to 10 minutes until flakes turn golden brown. Stir almond and coconut flakes once midway through roasting to prevent over-browning.
- Remove the baking sheet from the oven. Cool almond and coconut flakes for at least 10 minutes before sprinkling in cinnamon powder and salt. Toss to combine. Set aside.

Nutrition:

Calories: 62 kcal

Protein: 2.24 g

Fat: 4.01 g

Carbohydrates: 4.46 g

Bake Apple Turnover

Preparation Time: 30 minutes

Cooking Time: 25 minutes

Servings: 4

Ingredients:

1. For the turnovers
2. 4 apples, peeled, cored, diced into bite-sized pieces
3. 1 Tbsp. almond flour
4. All-purpose flour, for rolling out the dough
5. 1 frozen puff pastry, thawed
6. ½ cup palm sugar, crumbled by hand to loosen granules
7. ½ tsp. cinnamon powder
8. For the egg wash
9. 1 egg white, whisked in
10. 2 Tbsp. water

Directions:

- For the filling: combine almond flour, cinnamon powder, and palm sugar until these resemble coarse meal. Toss in diced apples until well coated. Set aside.

- On a lightly floured surface, roll the puff pastry until ¼ inch thin. Slice into 8 pieces of 4" x 4" squares.
- Divide prepared apples into 8 equal portions. Spoon on individual puff pastry squares. Fold in half diagonally. Press edges to seal.
- Place each filled pastry on a baking tray lined with parchment paper. Make sure there is ample space between pastries.
- Freeze for at least 20 minutes, or till ready to bake.
- Preheat oven to 400°F or 205°C for at 10 minutes.
- Brush frozen pastries with egg wash. Bring in a hot oven, and cook for 12 to 15 minutes, or until these turn golden brown all over.
- Take off the baking tray in the oven immediately. Cool slightly for easier handling.
- Place 1 apple turnover on a plate. Serve warm.

Nutrition:

Calories: 203 kcal,Protein: 5.29 g,Fat: 4.4 g
Carbohydrates: 38.25 g

Quinoa and Cauliflower Congee

Preparation Time: 10 minutes

Cooking Time: 1 hour

Servings: 8

Ingredients:

- 1 cauliflower head, minced
- 2 tablespoons red quinoa
- 2 leeks, minced
- 1 tablespoon fresh ginger, grated
- 2 garlic cloves, grated
- 6 cups of water
- 2 tablespoons brown rice
- 1 tablespoon olive oil
- 1 tablespoon fish sauce
- 2 onions, minced
- Pinch of white pepper
- For Garnish
- 4 eggs, soft-boiled
- 2 red chili, minced
- 1 lime, sliced into wedges
- ¼ cup packed basil leaves, torn
- ¼ cup loosely packed cilantro leaves, torn
- ¼ cup loosely packed spearmint leaves, torn

Directions:

1. Put olive oil into a huge skillet on medium heat. Sauté shallots, garlic, and ginger until limp and aromatic; pour into a slow cooker set at medium heat.
2. Except for garnishes, pour remaining ingredients into slow cooker; stir. Put the lid on. Cook for 6 hours. Turn off heat. Taste; adjust seasoning if needed.
3. Ladle congee into individual bowls. Garnish with basil leaves, cilantro leaves, red chilli, and spearmint leaves. Add 1 piece of soft-boiled egg on top of each; serve with a wedge of lime on the side. Slice egg just before eating so yolk runs into congee. Squeeze lime juice into congee just before eating.

Nutrition:

Calories: 138 kcal

Protein: 7.23 g

Fat: 7.65 g, Carbohydrates: 10.76 g

Breakfast Arrozcaldo

Preparation Time: 20 minutes

Cooking Time: 30 minutes

Servings: 5

Ingredients:

1. 6 eggs, white only
2. 1½ cups brown rice, cooked
3. For the filling
4. ¼ cup raisins
5. ½ cup frozen peas, thawed
6. 1 white onion, minced
7. 1 garlic clove, minced
8. oil, for greasing

Directions:

- For the filling, spray a small amount of oil into a skillet set over medium heat. Add in onion and garlic. Stir-fry until former is limp and transparent.

- Stir-fry while breaking up clumps, about 2 minutes. Add in remaining ingredients. Stir-fry for another minute.

- Turn down the heat, and let filling cook for 10 to 15 minutes, or until juices are greatly reduced. Stir often. Turn off heat. Divide into 6 equal portions.

- For the eggs, spray a small amount of oil into a smaller skillet set over medium heat. Cook eggs. Discard yolk. Transfer to holding the plate.
- To serve, place 1 portion of rice on a plate, 1 portion of filling, and 1 egg white. Serve warm.

Nutrition:

Calories: 53 kcal

Protein: 6.28 g

Fat: 1.35 g

Carbohydrates: 3.59 g

Apple Bruschetta with Almonds and Blackberries

Preparation Time: 20 minutes

Cooking Time: 30 minutes

Servings: 5

Ingredients:

1. 1 apple, sliced into ¼-inch thick half-moons
2. ¼ cup blackberries, thawed, lightly mashed
3. ½ tsp. fresh lemon juice
4. 1/8 cup almond slivers, toasted
5. Sea salt

Directions:

- Drizzle lemon juice on apple slices. Put these on a tray lined with parchment paper.
- Spread a small number of mashed berries on top of each slice. Top these off with the desired amount of almond slivers.
- Sprinkle sea salt on "bruschetta" just before serving.

Nutrition:

Calories: 56 kcal,Protein: 1.53 g,Fat: 1.43 g,Carbohydrates: 9.87 g

Hash Browns

Preparation Time: 15 minutes

Cooking Time: 15 minutes

Servings: 4

Ingredients:

1. 1 pound Russet potatoes, peeled, processed using a grater
2. Pinch of sea salt
3. Pinch of black pepper, to taste
4. 3 Tbsp. olive oil

Directions:

- Line a microwave safe-dish with paper towels. Spread shredded potatoes on top. Microwave veggies on the highest heat setting for 2 minutes. Remove from heat.
- Pour 1 tablespoon of oil into a non-stick skillet set over medium heat.
- Cooking in batches, place a generous pinch of potatoes into the hot oil. Press down using the back of a spatula.
- Cook for 3 minutes every side, or until brown and crispy. Drain on paper towels. Repeat step for remaining potatoes. Add more oil as needed.
- Season with salt and pepper. Serve.

Nutrition:

Calories:

200 kcal

Protein: 4.03 g

Fat: 11.73 g

Carbohydrates: 20.49 g

Sun-Dried Tomato Garlic Bruschetta

Preparation Time: 10 minutes

Cooking Time: 5 minutes

Servings: 6

Ingredients:

1. 2 slices sourdough bread, toasted
2. 1 tsp. chives, minced
3. 1 garlic clove, peeled
4. 2 tsp. sun-dried tomatoes in olive oil, minced
5. 1 tsp. olive oil

Directions:

- Vigorously rub garlic clove on 1 side of each of the toasted bread slices
- Spread equal portions of sun-dried tomatoes on the garlic side of bread. Sprinkle chives and drizzle olive oil on top.
- Pop both slices into oven toaster, and cook until well heated through.
- Place bruschetta on a plate. Serve warm.

Nutrition:

Calories: 149 kcal

Protein: 6.12 g

Fat: 2.99 g

Carbohydrates: 24.39 g

Mushroom Crêpes

Preparation Time: 1 hour 30 minutes

Cooking Time: 30 minutes

Servings: 6

Ingredients:

1. 2 eggs
2. 3/4 cup milk
3. 1/2 cup all-purpose flour
4. 1/4 teaspoon salt
5. For the filling
6. 3 tablespoons all-purpose flour
7. 2 cups of cremini mushrooms, sliced
8. 3/4 cup chicken broth
9. 1/2 cup Parmesan cheese, grated
10. 1/8 teaspoon cayenne
11. 1/8 teaspoon nutmeg
12. ¾ cup milk
13. 3 garlic cloves, minced
14. 2 tablespoons of parsley (chopped)
15. 6 slices of deli-sliced cooked lean ham
16. 1/4 teaspoon of salt
17. Freshly ground pepper

Directions:

- Put and combine the salt and flour in a bowl. In another bowl, whisk the eggs and milk. Gradually combine the two mixtures until smooth. Leave for 15 minutes.
- Spray a skillet using non-stick cooking spray and put over medium heat. Stir the batter a little. Add 1/4 of the batter into the skillet. Tilt the skillet to form a thin and even crêpe. Cook for 1-2 minutes or until the bottom is golden and the top is set. Flip and cook for 20 seconds. Transfer to a plate.
- Repeat the steps with the remaining batter. Loosely cover the cooked crêpes with plastic wrap.
- For the filling. Put all together the ingredients for filling in a saucepan on medium heat – flour, milk, cayenne, nutmeg, and pepper. Constantly whisk until thick or around 7 minutes. Remove from the stove. Stir in a tablespoon of parsley and cheese. Loosely cover to keep warm.
- Spray a skillet using non-stick cooking spray and put over medium heat. Cook the garlic and mushrooms. Season with salt. Cook for 6 minutes or until the mushrooms are soft. Add 2 tablespoons of sherry. Cook for a couple of minutes. Remove from the stove. Add the remaining parsley and stir.

- Put the crêpes side by side on a flat surface. Spread a tablespoon of the sauce and 2 tablespoons of the cooked mushrooms. Roll up the crêpes and transfer them to a greased baking dish. Put all the sauce on top. Bake in the oven at 450°F for 15 minutes.

Nutrition:

Calories: 232 kcal

Protein: 16.51 g

Fat: 10.8 g

Carbohydrates: 16.25 g

Oat Porridge with Cherry & Coconut

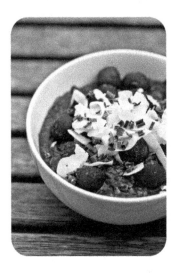

Preparation Time: 10 minutes

Cooking Time: 0 minutes

Servings: 3

Ingredients:

1. 1 ½ cups regular oats
2. 3 cups coconut milk
3. 4 tbsp. chia seed
4. 3 tbsp. raw cacao
5. Coconut shavings
6. Dark chocolate shavings
7. Fresh or frozen tart cherries
8. A pinch of stevia, optional
9. Maple syrup, to taste (optional)

Directions:

- Combine the oats, milk, stevia, and cacao in a medium saucepan over medium heat and bring to a boil. Lower the heat, then simmer until the oats are cooked to desired doneness.
- Divide the porridge among 3 serving bowls and top with dark chocolate and coconut shavings, cherries, and a little drizzle of maple syrup.

Nutrition:

Calories: 343 kcal

Protein: 15.64 g

Fat: 12.78 g

Carbohydrates: 41.63 g

Gingerbread Oatmeal Breakfast

Preparation Time: 10 minutes

Cooking Time: 0 minutes

Servings: 4

Ingredients:

1. 1 cup steel-cut oats
2. 4 cups drinking water
3. Organic Maple syrup, to taste
4. 1 tsp ground cloves
5. 1 ½ tbsp. ground cinnamon
6. 1/8 tsp nutmeg
7. ¼ tsp ground ginger
8. ¼ tsp ground coriander
9. ¼ tsp ground allspice
10. ¼ tsp ground cardamom
11. Fresh mixed berries

Directions:

- Cook the oats based on the package instructions. When it comes to a boil, reduce heat and simmer.
- Stir in all the spices and continue cooking until cooked to desired doneness.
- Serve in four serving bowls and drizzle with maple syrup and top with fresh berries.
- Enjoy!

Nutrition:

Calories: 87 kcal

Protein: 5.82 g

Fat: 3.26 g

Carbohydrates: 18.22 g

Apple, Ginger, and Rhubarb Muffins

Preparation Time: 15 minutes

Cooking Time: 25 minutes

Servings: 4

Ingredients:

- ½ cup finely ground almonds
- ¼ cup brown rice flour
- ½ cup buckwheat flour
- 1/8 cup unrefined raw sugar
- 2 tbsp. arrowroot flour
- 1 tbsp. linseed meal
- 2 tbsp. crystallized ginger, finely chopped
- ½ tsp. ground ginger
- ½ tsp. ground cinnamon
- 2 tsp. gluten-free baking powder
- A pinch of fine sea salt
- 1 small apple, peeled and finely diced
- 1 cup finely chopped rhubarb
- 1/3 cup almond/ rice milk
- 1 large egg
- ¼ cup extra virgin olive oil
- 1 tsp. pure vanilla extract

Directions:

- Set your oven to 350Fgrease an eight-cup muffin tin and line with paper cases.
- Combine the almond four, linseed meal, ginger and sugar in a mixing bowl. Sieve this mixture over the other flours, spices and baking powder and use a whisk to combine well.
- Stir in the apple and rhubarb in the flour mixture until evenly coated.
- In a separate bowl, whisk the milk, vanilla, and egg then pour it into the dry mixture. Stir until just combined – don't overwork the batter as this can yield very tough muffins.
- Scoop the mixture into the arrange muffin tin and top with a few slices of rhubarb. Bake for at least 25 minutes, till they start turning golden or when an inserted toothpick emerges clean.
- Take off from the oven and let sit for at least 5 minutes before transferring the muffins to a wire rack for further cooling.
- Serve warm with a glass of squeezed juice.
- Enjoy!

Nutrition:

Calories: 325 kcal

Protein: 6.32 g

Fat: 9.82 g

Carbohydrates: 55.71 g

Anti-Inflammatory Breakfast Frittata

Preparation Time: 10 minutes

Cooking Time: 40 minutes

Servings: 4

Ingredients:

1. 4 large eggs
2. 6 egg whites
3. 450g button mushrooms
4. 450g baby spinach
5. 125g firm tofu
6. 1 onion, chopped
7. 1 tbsp. minced garlic
8. ½ tsp. ground turmeric
9. ½ tsp. cracked black pepper
10. ¼ cup water
11. Kosher salt to taste

Directions:

1. Set your oven to 350F.
2. Sauté the mushrooms in a little bit of extra virgin olive oil in a large non-stick ovenproof pan over medium heat. Add the onions once the mushrooms start turning golden and cook for 3 minutes until the onions become soft.

3. Stir in the garlic then cook for at least 30 seconds until fragrant before adding the spinach. Pour in water, cover, and cook until the spinach becomes wilted for about 2 minutes.
4. Take off the lid and continue cooking up to the water evaporates. Now, combine the eggs, egg whites, tofu, pepper, turmeric, and salt in a bowl. When all the liquid has evaporated, pour in the egg mixture, let cook for about 2 minutes until the edges start setting, then transfer to the oven and bake for about 25 minutes or until cooked.
5. Take off from the oven then let sit for at least 5 minutes before cutting it into quarters and serving.
6. Enjoy!
7. Baby spinach and mushrooms boost the nutrient profile of the eggs to provide you with amazing anti-inflammatory benefits.

Nutrition:

Calories: 521 kcal

Protein: 29.13 g

Fat: 10.45 g

Carbohydrates: 94.94 g

Breakfast Sausage and Mushroom Casserole

Preparation Time: 20 minutes

Cooking Time: 45 minutes

Servings: 4

Ingredients:

- 450g of Italian sausage, cooked and crumbled
- Three-fourth cup of coconut milk
- 8 ounces of white mushrooms, sliced
- 1 medium onion, finely diced
- 2 Tablespoons of organic ghee
- 6 free-range eggs
- 600g of sweet potatoes
- 1 red bell pepper, roasted
- 3/4 tsp. of ground black pepper, divided
- 1 ½ tsp. of sea salt, divided

Directions:

- Peel and shred the sweet potatoes.
- Take a bowl, fill it with ice-cold water, and soak the sweet potatoes in it. Set aside.
- Peel the roasted bell pepper, remove its seeds and finely dice it.
- Set the oven 375°F.

- Get a casserole baking dish and grease it with the organic ghee.
- Put a skillet over medium flame and cook the mushrooms in it. Cook until the mushrooms are crispy and brown.
- Take the mushrooms out and mix them with the crumbled sausage.
- Now sauté the onions in the same skillet. Cook up to the onions are soft and golden. This should take about 4 – 5 minutes.
- Take the onions out and mix them in the sausage-mushroom mixture.
- Add the diced bell pepper to the same mixture.
- Mix well and set aside for a while.
- Now drain the soaked shredded potatoes, put them on a paper towel, and pat dry.
- Bring the sweet potatoes in a bowl and add about a teaspoon of salt and half a teaspoon of ground black pepper to it. Mix well and set aside.
- Now take a large bowl and crack the eggs in it.
- Break the eggs and then blend in the coconut milk.
- Stir in the remaining black pepper and salt.

- Take the greased casserole dish and spread the seasoned sweet potatoes evenly in the base of the dish.
- Next, spread the sausage mixture evenly in the dish.
- Finally, spread the egg mixture.
- Now cover the casserole dish using a piece of aluminum foil.
- Bake for 20 - 30 minutes. To check if the casserole is baked properly, insert a tester in the middle of the casserole, and it should come out clean.
- Uncover the casserole dish and bake it again, uncovered for 5 - 10 minutes, until the casserole is a little golden on the top.
- Allow it to cool for 10 minutes.
- Enjoy!

Nutrition:

Calories: 598 kcal

Protein: 28.65 g

Fat: 36.75 g

Carbohydrates: 48.01 g

Yummy Steak Muffins

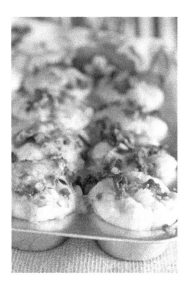

Preparation Time: 10 minutes

Cooking Time: 20 minutes

Servings: 4

Ingredients:

- 1 cup red bell pepper, diced
- 2 Tablespoons of water
- 8 ounce thin steak, cooked and finely chopped
- ¼ teaspoon of sea salt
- Dash of freshly ground black pepper
- 8 free-range eggs
- 1 cup of finely diced onion

Directions:

- Set the oven to 350°F
- Take 8 muffin tins and line then with parchment paper liners.
- Get a large bowl and crack all the eggs in it.
- Beat well the eggs.
- Blend in all the remaining ingredients.
- Spoon the batter into the arrange muffin tins. Fill three-fourth of each tin.
- Put the muffin tins in the preheated oven for about 20 minutes, until the muffins are baked and set in the middle.
- Enjoy!

Nutrition:

Calories: 151 kcal

Protein: 17.92 g

Fat: 7.32 g

Carbohydrates: 3.75 g

White and Green Quiche

Preparation Time: 10 minutes

Cooking Time: 40 minutes

Servings: 3

Ingredients:

1. 3 cups of fresh spinach, chopped
2. 15 large free-range eggs
3. 3 cloves of garlic, minced
4. 5 white mushrooms, sliced
5. 1 small sized onion, finely chopped
6. 1 ½ teaspoon of baking powder
7. Ground black pepper to taste
8. 1 ½ cups of coconut milk
9. Ghee, as required to grease the dish
10. Sea salt to taste

Directions:

- Set the oven to 350°F.
- Get a baking dish then grease it with the organic ghee.
- Break all the eggs in a huge bowl then whisk well.
- Stir in coconut milk. Beat well
- While you are whisking the eggs, start adding the remaining ingredients in it.

- When all the ingredients are thoroughly blended, pour all of it into the prepared baking dish.
- Bake for at least 40 minutes, up to the quiche is set in the middle.
- Enjoy!

Nutrition:

Calories: 608 kcal

Protein: 20.28 g

Fat: 53.42 g

Carbohydrates: 16.88 g

Beef Breakfast Casserole

Preparation Time: 10 minutes

Cooking Time: 30 minutes

Servings: 5

Ingredients:

1. 1 pound of ground beef, cooked
2. 10 eggs
3. ½ cup Pico de Gallo
4. 1 cup baby spinach
5. ¼ cup sliced black olives
6. Freshly ground black pepper

Directions:

- Preheat oven to 350 degrees Fahrenheit. Prepare a 9" glass pie plate with non-stick spray.
- Whisk the eggs until frothy. Season with salt and pepper.
- Layer the cooked ground beef, Pico de Gallo, and spinach in the pie plate.
- Slowly pour the eggs over the top.
- Top with black olives.
- Bake for at least 30 minutes, until firm in the middle.
- Slice into 5 pieces and serve.

Nutrition:

Calories: 479 kcal

Protein: 43.54 g

Fat: 30.59 g

Carbohydrates: 4.65 g

Ham and Veggie Frittata Muffins

Preparation Time: 10 minutes

Cooking Time: 25 minutes

Servings: 12

Ingredients:

1. 5 ounces thinly sliced ham
2. 8 large eggs
3. 4 tablespoons coconut oil
4. ½ yellow onion, finely diced
5. 8 oz. frozen spinach, thawed and drained
6. 8 oz. mushrooms, thinly sliced
7. 1 cup cherry tomatoes, halved
8. ¼ cup coconut milk (canned)
9. 2 tablespoons coconut flour
10. Sea salt and pepper to taste

Directions:

- Preheat oven to 375 degrees Fahrenheit.
- In a medium skillet, warm the coconut oil on medium heat. Add the onion and cook until softened.
- Add the mushrooms, spinach, and cherry tomatoes. Season with salt and pepper. Cook until the mushrooms have softened. About 5 minutes. Remove from heat and set aside.

- In a huge bowl, beat the eggs together with the coconut milk and coconut flour. Stir in the cooled the veggie mixture.
- Line each cavity of a 12 cavity muffin tin with the thinly sliced ham. Pour the egg mixture into each one and bake for 20 minutes.
- Remove from oven and allow to cool for about 5 minutes before transferring to a wire rack.
- To maximize the benefit of a vegetable-rich diet, it's important to eat a variety of colors, and these veggie-packed frittata muffins do just that. The onion, spinach, mushrooms, and cherry tomatoes provide a wide range of vitamins and nutrients and a healthy dose of fiber.

Nutrition:

Calories: 125 kcal

Protein: 5.96 g

Fat: 9.84 g

Carbohydrates: 4.48 g

Tomato and Avocado Omelet

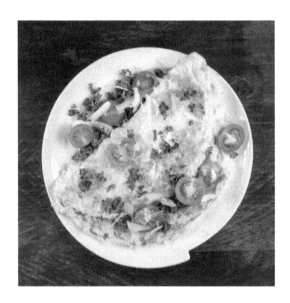

Preparation Time: 5 minutes

Cooking Time: 5 minutes

Servings: 1

Ingredients:

1. 2 eggs
2. ¼ avocado, diced
3. 4 cherry tomatoes, halved
4. 1 tablespoon cilantro, chopped
5. Squeeze of lime juice
6. Pinch of salt

Directions:

- Put together the avocado, tomatoes, cilantro, lime juice, and salt in a small bowl, then mix well and set aside.
- Warm a medium nonstick skillet on medium heat. Whisk the eggs until frothy and add to the pan. Move the eggs around gently with a rubber spatula until they begin to set.
- Scatter the avocado mixture over half of the omelet. Remove from heat, and slide the omelet onto a plate as you fold it in half.
- Serve immediately.

Nutrition:

Calories: 433 kcal

Protein: 25.55 g

Fat: 32.75 g

Carbohydrates: 10.06 g

Vegan-Friendly Banana Bread

Preparation Time: 15 minutes

Cooking Time: 40 minutes

Servings: 4-6

Ingredients:

1. 2 ripe bananas, mashed
2. 1/3 cup brewed coffee
3. 3 tbsp. chia seeds
4. 6 tbsp. water
5. ½ cup soft vegan butter
6. ½ cup maple syrup
7. 2 cups flour
8. 2 tsp. baking powder
9. 1 tsp. cinnamon powder
10. 1 tsp. allspice
11. ½ tsp. salt

Directions:

- Set oven at 350F.
- Bring the chia seeds in a small bowl then soak it with 6 tbsp. of water. Stir well and set aside.
- In a mixing bowl, mix using a hand mixer the vegan butter and maple syrup until it turns fluffy. Add the chia seeds along with the mashed bananas.
- Mix well and then add the coffee.

- Meanwhile, sift all the dry ingredients (flour, baking powder, cinnamon powder, all spice, and salt) and then gradually add into the bowl with the wet ingredients.
- Combine the ingredients well and then pour over a baking pan lined with parchment paper.
- Place in the oven to bake for at least 30-40 minutes, or until the toothpick comes out clean after inserting in the bread.
- Allow the bread to cool before serving.

Nutrition:

Calories: 371 kcal

Protein: 5.59 g

Fat: 16.81 g

Carbohydrates: 49.98 g

Mango Granola

Preparation Time: 10 minutes

Cooking Time: 30 minutes

Servings: 4

Ingredients:

1. 2 cups rolled oats
2. 1 cup dried mango, chopped
3. ½ cup almonds, roughly chopped
4. ½ cup nuts
5. ½ cup dates, roughly chopped
6. 3 tbsp. sesame seeds
7. 2 tsp. cinnamon
8. 2/3 cup agave nectar
9. 2 tbsp. coconut oil
10. 2 tbsp. water

Directions:

- Set oven at 320F
- In a large bowl, put the oats, almonds, nuts, sesame seeds, dates, and cinnamon then mix well.
- Meanwhile, heat a saucepan over medium heat, pour in the agave syrup, coconut oil, and water.
- Stir and let it cook for at least 3 minutes or until the coconut oil has melted.

- Gradually pour the syrup mixture into the bowl with the oats and nuts and stir well, ensure that all the ingredients are coated with the syrup.
- Transfer the granola on a baking sheet lined with parchment paper and place in the oven to bake for 20 minutes.
- After 20 minutes, take off the tray from the oven and lay the chopped dried mango on top. Put back in the oven then bake again for another 5 minutes.
- Let the granola cool to room temperature before serving or placing it in an airtight container for storage. The shelf life of the granola will last up to 2-3 weeks.

Nutrition:

Calories: 434 kcal

Protein: 13.16 g

Fat: 28.3 g

Carbohydrates: 55.19 g

Sautéed Veggies on Hot Bagels

Preparation Time: 10 minutes

Cooking Time: 16 minutes

Servings: 2

Ingredients:

1. 1 yellow squash, diced
2. 1 zucchini, sliced thin
3. ½ onion, sliced thin
4. 2 pcs. tomatoes, sliced
5. 1 clove of garlic, chopped
6. salt and pepper to taste
7. 1 tbsp. olive oil
8. 2 pcs. vegan bagels
9. vegan butter for spread

Directions:

- Heat the olive oil on the medium temperature in a cast-iron skillet.
- Lower the heat to medium-low and sauté the onions for 10 minutes or until the onions start to brown.
- Turn the heat again to medium and then add the diced squash and zucchini to the pan and cook for 5 minutes. Add the clove of garlic and cook for another minute.

- Throw in the tomato slices to the pan and cook for 1 minute. Season with pepper and salt and turn off the heat.
- Toast the bagels and cut in half.
- Spread the bagels lightly with butter and serve with the sautéed veggies on top.

Nutrition:

Calories: 375 kcal

Protein: 14.69 g

Fat: 11.46 g

Carbohydrates: 54.61 g

Coco-Tapioca Bowl

Preparation Time: 10 minutes

Cooking Time: 20 minutes

Servings: 2

Ingredients:

1. ¼ cup tapioca pearls, small sized
2. 1 can light coconut milk
3. ¼ cup maple syrup
4. 1 ½ tsp. lemon juice
5. ½ cup unsweetened coconut flakes, toasted
6. 2 cups water

Directions:

- Place the tapioca in a saucepan and pour over the 2 cups of water. Let it stand for at least 30 minutes.
- Pour in the coconut milk and syrup and heat the saucepan over medium temperature. Bring to a boil while stirring constantly.
- Add the lemon juice and stir and then garnish with coconut flakes.

Nutrition:

Calories: 309 kcal

Protein: 3.93 g

Fat: 9.02 g

Carbohydrates: 54.55 g

Choco-Banana Oats

Preparation Time: 5 minutes

Cooking Time: 8 minutes

Servings: 2

Ingredients:

1. 2 cups oats
2. 2 cups almond milk
3. ¾ cup water
4. 2 ripe bananas, sliced
5. ¼ tsp. Vanilla
6. ¼ tsp. almond extract
7. 2 tbsp. cocoa powder, unsweetened
8. 2 tbsp. agave nectar
9. 1/8 tsp. cinnamon
10. 1/8 tsp. salt
11. 1/3 cup toasted walnuts, chopped
12. 2 tbsp. vegan chocolate chips, semisweet

Directions:

- In a large saucepan, pour the almond milk, water, bananas, vanilla, and almond extract. Add the salt, stir, and heat over high temperature.
- Mix the oats in the pan along with the unsweetened cocoa powder, 1 tbsp. agave nectar and lower the temperature to medium. Cook for 7-8 minutes, or

until the oats are cooked to your liking. Stir frequently.

- Scoop the cooked oats into serving bowls and garnish with the chopped walnuts, chocolate chips, and drizzle with the remaining agave nectar.

Nutrition:

Calories: 522 kcal

Protein: 30.17 g

Fat: 27.01 g

Carbohydrates: 79.09 g

Savory Bread

Preparation Time: 10 minutes

Cooking Time: 20-25 minutes

Servings: 8-10

Ingredients:

1. ½ cup plus 1tablespoon almond flour
2. 1 tsp. baking soda
3. 1 teaspoon ground turmeric
4. Salt, to taste
5. 2 large organic eggs
6. 2 organic egg whites
7. 1 cup raw cashew butter
8. 1 tablespoon water
9. 1 tablespoon apple cider vinegar

Directions:

- Set the oven to 350F. Grease a loaf pan.
- In a big pan, mix together flour, baking soda, turmeric, and salt.
- In another bowl, add eggs, egg whites, and cashew butter and beat till smooth.
- Gradually, add water and beat till well combined.
- Add flour mixture and mix till well combined.
- Stir in apple cider vinegar treatment.
- Place a combination into prepared loaf pan evenly.

- Bake for around twenty minutes or till a toothpick inserted within the center is released clean.

Nutrition:

Calories: 347

Fat: 11g

Carbohydrates: 29g

Fiber: 6g

Protein: 21g

Savory Veggie Muffins

Preparation Time: 15 minutes

Cooking Time: 18-23 minutes

Servings: 5

Ingredients:

1. ¾ cup almond meal
2. ½ tsp baking soda
3. ¼ cup concentrate powder
4. 2 teaspoons fresh dill, chopped
5. Salt, to taste
6. 4 large organic eggs
7. 1½ tablespoons nutritional yeast
8. 2 teaspoons apple cider vinegar
9. 3 tablespoons fresh lemon juice
10. 2 tablespoons coconut oil, melted
11. 1 cup coconut butter, softened
12. 1 bunch scallion, chopped
13. 2 medium carrots, peeled and grated
14. ½ cup fresh parsley, chopped

Directions:

- Set the oven to 350F. Grease 10 cups of your large muffin tin.
- In a large bowl, mix together flour, baking soda, Protein powder, and salt.

- In another bowl, add eggs, nutritional yeast, vinegar, lemon juice, and oil and beat till well combined.
- Add coconut butter and beat till the mixture becomes smooth.
- Put egg mixture into the flour mixture and mix till well combined.
- Fold in scallion, carts, and parsley.
- Place the amalgamation into prepared muffin cups evenly.
- Bake for about 18-23 minutes or till a toothpick inserted inside center comes out clean.

Nutrition:

Calories: 378

Fat: 13g

Carbohydrates: 32g

Fiber: 11g

Protein: 32g

Crepes with Coconut Cream & Strawberry Sauce

Preparation Time: 15 minutes

Cooking Time: 8 minutes

Servings: 4

Ingredients:

1. For Sauce:
2. 12-ounces frozen strawberries, thawed and liquid reserved
3. 1½ teaspoons tapioca starch
4. 1 tablespoon honey
5. For the Coconut cream:
6. 1 (13½-ounce) can chilled coconut milk
7. 1 teaspoon organic vanilla flavoring
8. 1 tablespoon organic honey
9. For Crepes:
10. 2 tablespoons tapioca starch
11. 2 tablespoons coconut flour
12. ¼ cup almond milk
13. 2 organic eggs
14. Pinch of salt
15. Avocado oil, as required

Directions:

- For sauce inside a bowl, mix together some reserved strawberry liquid and tapioca starch.
- Add remaining ingredients and mix well.
- Transfer a combination inside a pan on medium-high heat.
- Bring to a boil, stirring continuously.
- Cook for at least 2-3 minutes, till the sauce, becomes thick.
- Remove from heat and aside, covered till serving.
- For coconut cream, carefully, scoop your cream from your surface of a can of coconut milk.
- In a mixer, add coconut cream, vanilla flavoring, and honey and pulse for around 6-8 minutes or till fluffy.
- For crepes in a blender, add all ingredients and pulse till well combined and smooth.
- Lightly, grease a substantial nonstick skillet with avocado oil as well as heat on medium-low heat.
- Add a modest amount of mixture and tilt the pan to spread it evenly inside the skillet.
- Cook approximately 1-2 minutes.
- Carefully change the side and cook for approximately 1-1½ minutes more.
- Repeat with the remaining mixture.

- Divide the coconut cream onto each crepe evenly and fold into quarters.
- Place strawberry sauce ahead and serve.

Nutrition:

Calories: 364

Fat: 9g

Carbohydrates: 26g

Fiber: 7g

Protein: 15g

Spicy Ginger Crepes

Preparation Time: 15 minutes

Cooking Time: 20-30 seconds

Servings: 8

Ingredients:

1. 1 1/3 cups chickpea flour
2. ½ teaspoon red chili powder
3. Salt, to taste
4. 1 (1-inch) fresh ginger piece, grated finely
5. 1 cup fresh cilantro leaves, chopped
6. 1 green chili, seeded and chopped finely
7. 1 cup water
8. Cooking spray, as required

Directions:

- In a sizable bowl, mix together flour, chili powder, and salt.
- Add ginger, cilantro, and chili and mix well.
- Add water and mix till an even mixture form.
- Keep aside, covered for approximately ½-120 minutes.
- Lightly, grease a substantial nonstick skillet with cooking spray and heat on medium-high heat.
- Add the desired volume of the mixture and tilt the pan to spread it evenly inside the skillet.

- Cook approximately 10-15 seconds per side.
- Repeat while using the remaining mixture.

Nutrition:

Calories: 73

Fat: 1.3

Carbohydrates: 11g

Fiber: 2.1g,

Protein: 4.3g

Honey Pancakes

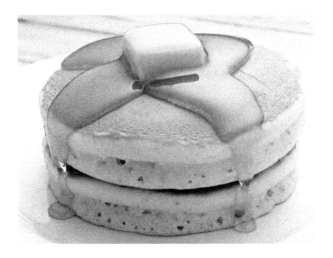

Preparation Time: 10 minutes

Cooking Time: 5 minutes

Servings: 2

Ingredients:

1. ½ cup almond flour
2. 2 tablespoons coconut flour
3. 1 tablespoon ground flaxseeds
4. ¼ tsp baking soda
5. ½ tablespoon ground ginger
6. ½ tablespoon ground nutmeg
7. ½ tablespoon ground cinnamon
8. ½ teaspoon ground cloves
9. Pinch of salt

10. 2 tablespoons organic honey

11. ¾ cup organic egg whites

12. ½ teaspoon organic vanilla extract

13. Coconut oil, as required

Directions:

- In a big bowl, mix together flours, flax seeds, baking soda, spices, and salt.
- In another bowl, add honey, egg whites and vanilla and beat till well combined.
- Put the egg mixture into the flour mixture then mix till well combined.
- Lightly, grease a big nonstick skillet with oil and heat on medium-low heat.
- Add about ¼ cup of mixture and tilt the pan to spread it evenly inside the skillet.
- Cook for about 3-4 minutes.
- Carefully, customize the side and cook approximately 1 minute more.
- Repeat with the remaining mixture.
- Serve along with your desired topping.

Nutrition:

Calories: 291

Fat: 8g

Carbohydrates: 26g

Fiber: 4g,Protein: 23g

Cilantro Pancakes

Preparation Time: 10 minutes

Cooking Time: 6-8 minutes

Servings: 6

Ingredients:

1. ½ cup tapioca flour
2. ½ cup almond flour
3. ½ teaspoon chili powder
4. ¼ teaspoon ground turmeric
5. Salt, to taste
6. Freshly ground black pepper, to taste
7. 1 cup full- fat coconut milk
8. ½ of red onion, chopped
9. 1 (½-inch) fresh ginger piece, grated finely
10. 1 Serrano pepper, minced
11. ½ cup fresh cilantro, chopped
12. Oil, as required

Directions:

- In a big bowl, put together the flours and spices then mix.
- Put the coconut milk and mix till well combined.
- Fold within the onion, ginger, Serrano pepper, and cilantro.

- Lightly, grease a sizable nonstick skillet with oil and warmth on medium-low heat.
- Add about ¼ cup of mixture and tilt the pan to spread it evenly inside the skillet.
- Cook for around 3-4 minutes from either side.
- Repeat with all the remaining mixture.
- Serve along with your desired topping.

Nutrition:

Calories: 331

Fat: 10g

Carbohydrates: 37g

Fiber: 6g

Protein: 28g

Zucchini Pancakes

Preparation Time: 15 minutes

Cooking Time: 6-10 min

Servings: 8

Ingredients:

1. 1 cup chickpea flour
2. 1½ cups water, divided
3. ¼ teaspoon cumin seeds
4. ¼ tsp cayenne
5. ¼ teaspoon ground turmeric
6. Salt, to taste
7. ½ cup zucchini, shredded
8. ½ cup red onion, chopped finely
9. 1 green chile, seeded and chopped finely
10. ¼ cup fresh cilantro, chopped

Directions:

- In a large bowl, add flour and ¾ cup with the water and beat till smooth.
- Add remaining water and beat till a thin
- Fold inside the onion, ginger, Serrano pepper, and cilantro.
- Lightly, grease a substantial nonstick skillet with oil and heat on medium-low heat.

- Add about ¼ cup of mixture and tilt the pan to spread it evenly in the skillet.
- Cook for around 4-6 minutes.
- Carefully, alter the side and cook for approximately 2-4 minutes.
- Repeat while using the remaining mixture.
- Serve together with your desired topping.

Nutrition:

Calories: 389

Fat: 13g

Carbohydrates: 25g

Fiber: 4g

Protein: 21g

Pumpkin & Banana Waffles

Preparation Time: 15 minutes

Cooking Time: 5 minutes

Servings: 4

Ingredients:

1. ½ cup almond flour
2. ½ cup coconut flour
3. 1 tsp baking soda
4. 1½ teaspoons ground cinnamon
5. ¾ teaspoon ground ginger
6. ½ teaspoon ground cloves
7. ½ teaspoon ground nutmeg
8. Salt, to taste
9. 2 tablespoons olive oil
10. 5 large organic eggs
11. ¾ cup almond milk
12. ½ cup pumpkin puree
13. 2 medium bananas, peeled and sliced

Directions:

- Preheat the waffle iron, and after that, grease it.
- In a sizable bowl, mix together flours, baking soda, and spices.
- In a blender, put the remaining ingredients and pulse till smooth.

- Add flour mixture and pulse till
- In preheated waffle iron, add the required quantity of mixture.
- Cook approximately 4-5 minutes.
- Repeat using the remaining mixture.

Nutrition:

Calories: 357.2

Fat: 28.5g

Carbohydrates: 19.7g

Fiber: 4g

Protein: 14g

Blueberry & Cashew Waffles

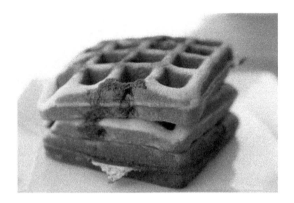

Preparation Time: 15 minutes

Cooking Time: 4-5 minutes

Servings: 5

Ingredients:

1. 1 cup raw cashews
2. 3 tablespoons coconut flour
3. 1 tsp baking soda
4. Salt, to taste
5. ½ cup unsweetened almond milk
6. 3 organic eggs
7. ¼ cup coconut oil, melted
8. 3 tablespoons organic honey
9. ½ teaspoon organic vanilla flavor
10. 1 cup fresh blueberries

Directions:

- Preheat the waffle iron after which grease it.
- In a mixer, add cashews and pulse till flour-like consistency forms.
- Transfer the cashew flour in a big bowl.
- Add almond flour, baking soda and salt and mix well.
- In another bowl, put the remaining ingredients and beat till well combined.
- Put the egg mixture into the flour mixture then mix till well combined.
- Fold in blueberries.
- In preheated waffle iron, add the required amount of mixture.
- Cook for around 4-5 minutes.
- Repeat with the remaining mixture.

Nutrition:

Calories: 432

Fat: 32

Carbohydrates: 32g

Protein: 13g

Cheddar and Chive Souffles

Preparation Time: 10 minutes

Cooking Time: 25 minutes

Servings: 8

Ingredients:

1. ½ cup almond flour
2. ¼ cup chopped chives
3. 1 tsp salt
4. ½ tsp xanthan gum
5. 1 tsp ground mustard
6. ¼ tsp cayenne pepper
7. ½ tsp cracked black pepper
8. ¾ cup heavy cream
9. 2 cups shredded cheddar cheese
10. ½ cup baking powder
11. 6 organic eggs, separated

Directions:

- Switch on the oven, then set its temperature to 350°F and let it preheat.
- Take a medium bowl, add flour in it, add remaining ingredients, except for baking powder and eggs, and whisk until combined.

- Separate egg yolks and egg whites between two bowls, add egg yolks in the flour mixture and whisk until incorporated.
- Add baking powder into the egg whites and beat with an electric mixer until stiff peaks form and then stir egg whites into the flour mixture until well mixed.
- Divide the batter evenly between eight ramekins and then bake for 25 minutes until done.
- Serve straight away or store in the refrigerator until ready to eat.

Nutrition:

Calories 288

Total Fat 21g

Total Carbs 3g

Protein 14g

Conclusion

The anti-inflammatory diet cookbook is the perfect resource for anyone who is suffering from inflammation. This cookbook has a special focus on reducing inflammation in the joints, cartilage, and muscles. Each recipe has been carefully developed to help reduce joint pain, joint stiffness, and even autoimmune disorders such as lupus and rheumatoid arthritis.

While most people associate food with comfort, a large number of foods are actually capable of having a dramatic impact on your health. Foods that are high in good fats (omega-3) are especially beneficial for many issues that affect the body. This cookbook provides recipes that are high in good fats and low in inflammatory foods like gluten and dairy. These recipes can be used to help create an anti-inflammatory diet that can help you feel better! The inflammatory disease will lead to many different health consequences and will even attack our most vital organs. The best way to do this is to prevent chronic inflammation in the first place. The next best thing is to recognize the signs and symptoms as early as possible, so proper interventions can be done to limit and reverse the impact of chronic inflammation. Inflammatory disease is the root cause of many long-term diseases, so ignoring the warning signs can create major consequences for your health.

Unfortunately, if the inflammatory disease gets out of control, preventative measures may be out of the question, and medical interventions will need to be done. Our goal is to prevent you from getting to this point. Lucky for us, many lifestyle changes can be performed to stop and reverse this disease process when it is still in its in advance stages. This is another reason why we should recognize and not ignore the signs and symptoms. A major lifestyle change we can commit to is a new diet plan. The anti-inflammatory diet is a meal plan that boasts healthy and nutritious cuisines, but still flavorful and appealing to the taste buds. There is a major myth out there that healthy food cannot be delicious. We have proven this myth wrong by providing numerous recipes from around the world that follow our healthy meal plan.

We hope that the information you read in this book gives you a better understanding of how the immune system functions and how a proper diet plan can help protect it and our other valuable cells and tissues. The recipes we have provided are just a starting point. Use them as a guide to create many of your dishes that follow the diet plan. Just make sure you use the proper ingredients and food groups.

Also, for maximum results, follow the Anti-Inflammatory Diet food Guide Pyramid.

The next step is to take the instruction we have provided and begin taking steps to change your life and improve your health. Begin recognizing the signs and symptoms of chronic inflammation and make the necessary lifestyle changes to prevent further health problems. Start transitioning to the anti-inflammatory diet today by incorporating small meals into your schedule and increase the amount as tolerated. Within a short period, the diet will be a regular part of your routine. You will notice increased energy, improved mental function, a stronger and well-balanced immune system, reduction in chronic pain, some healthy weight loss, and overall better health outcomes. If you are ready to experience these changes, then wait no longer and begin putting your knowledge from this book into action.

CPSIA information can be obtained
at www.ICGtesting.com
Printed in the USA
BVHW081957260421
605884BV00013B/377